NATURAL HAIR CARE GUIDE

HOW TO STOP HAIR LOSS AND ACCELERATE HAIR GROWTH IN A NATURAL WAY

GET STRONG, HEALTHY AND SHINY HAIR WITHOUT CHEMICALS

BY MIRANDA ROSS

TABLE OF CONTENTS

Introduction

I want to thank you and congratulate you for purchasing the book "Natural Hair Care Guide: How To Stop Hair Loss And Accelerate Hair Growth In A Natural Way, Get Strong, Healthy And Shiny Hair Without Chemicals".

There are many people, especially girls, who choose not to go out and socialize just because their hair isn't in the mood that day. Everyone is conscious when it comes to the look of their hair, especially if they are going to meet other people. Hair can make impressions on job interviews, date, night outs, etc.

Studies have shown that we begin to make an impression of the character and personality of a person within seconds after seeing them. While a big amount of aspects starting from makeup to clothing options also make an impact on the impressions we make, hairstyle have been shown to be one of the most renowned aspects in making an impression.

Hair care is extremely important for working individuals, particularly for the ones that are in the field of marketing and work together with clients and different kinds of people regularly. Beautiful hair gives us confidence and poise. People can carry themselves assertively in the presence of others, and their conclusive power grows; that why people with great personalities are chosen in marketing fields of a business.

Dry, dead, and dull hair not just hampers the personality but it outshines the person's skills as well. It's obvious that people who don't have soft, smooth, and shiny hair are averse to show off in public, and avoid being at places full of people. Also, their interaction abilities fade away and they lose their confidence.

There are a lot of shampoos, herbs, oils, and serums you can easily find in the market that guarantee to give shine and life to our hair. There are products guarantee that we will get results within a week or two while there are herbal products that give results steadily and slow but surely worth the wait.

In addition, ideal hair texture isn't everything. Styles of hair also define different personalities. People who choose to have short and stylish hair are known to be risk takers and more confident, while those who have long and smooth hair are seen to be more classic and simple.

Teenagers usually like to do experiment with their hair, but when it comes to the texture, everybody gets emotional and nobody bears dull and dead hair. There are different hairs styles are being introduced day by day; some like to cling to their old trademark of hair style while there are also some who likes changing it from time to time.

But at the end of the day, no matter what kind of style you want for your hair, the most important thing you have to learn is how to take care of it. In this book you will learn some natural hair care tips to keep your hair healthy and glowing.

The trademarks that are used are without any consent, and the publication of the trademark is without permission or backing by the trademark owner. All trademarks and brands within this book are for clarifying purposes only and are the owned by the owners themselves, not affiliated with this document.

DISCLAIMER: The purpose of this book is to provide information only. The information, though believed to be entirely accurate, is NOT a substitution for medical, psychological or professional advice, diagnosis or treatment. The author recommends that you seek the advice of your physician or other qualified health care provider to present them with questions you may have regarding any medical condition. Advice from your trusted, professional medical advisor should always supersede information presented in this book.

Chapter 1: 5 Most Common Hair Problems

Hair could be straight and short, wavy and long, shiny and smooth, or unmanageable and frizzy. Hair comes in different colors, lengths, styles, and textures. But almost everyone, despite the kinds they have, experiences some hair problems sometimes. Here are some of the most common problems people are facing when it comes to their hair:

Hair loss

The health conditions that usually lead to extreme hair loss include medications, serious infections, thyroid, surgical operations, hormonal imbalance, fungal infections, pregnancy, autoimmune sicknesses, and stress. When hair loss does something with medication, discontinuing medication stops further loss and gradually, it'll grow back to normal. Transplants could also be done to give you a lasting replacement solution.

Gray hair

There are people who think that that gray hair makes them look unique, while for most, it is a simple sign of aging. Having white or gray hair is very inevitable as people age. Scientists show hair stems its color from melanin, a color created by melanocyte cells that found in the hair follicles. Researchers say that the melanocytes sustain increasing damage as years go by that making them unable to produce melanin. The accumulation of the DNA and hydrogen peroxide damage are conceivable reasons for the commotion of the melanin fabrication.

Thinning Hair

Throughout the last 20 years, dermatologists have noticed a slow increase in the amount of people that are experiencing complications related to losing of hair. If you want to stop your hair in getting thinner, it's important to know the primary reasons why thinning hair happens and what peripheral factors might be triggering it. While genetic aspects play the utmost part in determining if a person is going go through thinning hair, there are also a lot of other aspects that could have a big part like diet, hair products, and others.

Dandruff

This hair problem is produced by the chemical reaction within the body that rises normal flaking of dead cells. The chemical reaction could be caused by stress, dietary deficiency, incorrect usage of hair products, and hormonal imbalance.

Brittle Hair

It's common for women to begin noticing that their hair becomes brittle and dry. It's usually an early sign that your hair is having some problems and it won't from there just yet. A hair quality loss might just be the reason for regular coloring doing hair treatments, but if you are not doing any of this and it still gets brittle, there is a great chance you are on the way to losing your hair.

Chapter 2: Natural Treatments For 5 Most Common Hair Problems

Hair Loss

The best thing about hair loss natural treatment is that it includes naturally made ingredients. Different from artificial hair loss treatments you can find in the market today, natural treatments do not contain any known damaging side effects.

You have to consider that there are researchers studying different types of herbs so as to find ways to prevent hair loss. In recent times, they discovered that there are many plants and herbs that can ultimately stop hair loss and even make hair regrow again.

To keep your hair healthy, you have to know that it have to be correctly nurtured. And to make this happen, the blood flow in your scalp have to be rich in nutrient.

You must also remember that there are many other factors that can lead to hair loss. It could be produced by diseases, emotional stress, environmental aspects, hormonal imbalance, thyroid, immune system conditions, and it could also be triggered by medication and your genetic factor.

Now, to treat hair loss, you'll notice that the right nutrition and the proper kinds of herbs can offer nourishment on the follicles of your hair that can revive it and begin growing hair once more. There are many herbs that are able to stop and help treat the losing of hair. Some of these are aloe vera, sesame oil, green tea, saw palmetto, and horsetail.

There are also herbs that you can consume or drink, while some are herbs that you are able to use externally. You can use the aloe vera to rinse your hair. Not just that it will keep your scalp in good shape but it will also stimulate the follicles of your hair.

Gray Hair

If you want to prevent your hair from turning gray, you just simply have to follow these simple steps. If you are smoker, then you have to consider quitting. Cigarette is one of the worst enemies of our body. Start eating healthy and have a balanced diet. Eat the right amount of eggs, meat, milk, fish, nuts, and other products filled with beneficial elements and vitamins for our body. You can use oil masks and other homemade oil at least few times a week.

You can also consider coloring dying your hair without using artificial products. The natural method of dying your hair is by coloring it using boiled tea leaves, with this you'll see the result a bit later and you may not get the shade you want, but it is so much safer for your skin and does not damage the hair.

Thinning Hair

Using hot oil massages is one of the best things you can do for thinning hair. You can massage your scalp for 15 minutes using hot mixture of two teaspoons olive oil and two teaspoons of coconut oil. After doing this, you can start wiping your hair using a towel soaked in hot water and then just let it dry. Do this for 2 or 3 times to get the better result and you can rinse the oils off your hair using natural shampoo.

Another type of oil you can use to naturally treat your thinning hair is the castor oil. You have to warm a cup of castor oil, scrub it all over your scalp and then comb your hair. Wrap your hair using a hot towel and wash the oil off using natural shampoo.

You can also treat your hair using olive oil and honey. Produce a mixture of a cup of olive oil and a cup of liquid honey and mix them well. Store the mixture for a few days and then use it on your scalp and hair. Comb your hair but make sure that the comb is not going to touch the scalp and then cover it with tight shower cap. Leave it for at least an hour then rinse it well.

Keep in mind that shampooing your hair regularly is advantageous to hair, but you have to be careful on your shampoo option. It is always better to use mild shampoos as stronger hair products can damage your hair. During the summer, you could only dampen your hair a bit on a daily basis and keep it conditioned that way. You are able to use rosemary water in place of using just water.

A natural protein treatment is also very beneficial. Mix an egg yolk with a teaspoon of olive oil and a teaspoon of vinegar. Leave it on your head for 10 to 15 minutes before rinsing it.

Nutrition is another thing to look at to, if you want to keep your hair from thinning. Protein consumption is needed for good hair growth because hair is completely made of protein. Foods that are great sources of protein are eggs, meat, green dhal, and soy. In addition to protein, your hair requires vitamins to grow beautifully.

Dandruff

There are primarily two different reasons why we are getting dandruffs – internal and external reasons. The internal reasons of dandruff are because of emotional stress, poor hygiene, excessive sugar, lack of rest, and too much fat in the diet. The external reasons are extreme hair sprays usage, infrequent use of shampoo, or dry indoor heating. Here are 6 useful natural dandruff treatments you can make and use at home:

- Coconut Oil with Camphor

Mix coconut or neem oil with a spoonful of camphor and massage the mixture on the scalp. This would be an efficient natural dandruff management.

- Hazel with Lemon

Mix one tablespoon lemon juice with 100g witch hazel. Add 200ml of water and then you can use this mixture in washing your hair. You can do it a lot of times until the hair becomes dandruff free.

- Olive oil and almond oil

Mix olive oil and almond oil. Massage the mixture on your scalp and let it on your scalp for good 5 minutes. Wash thoroughly.

- Pain Killer with Shampoo

13

Crush two tablets of aspirins and mix it with mild shampoo. Apply it over the scalp and leave it for about 2 minutes. Wash until all the aspirin residues from the hair gets removed.

- Glycerin with coconut oil

Mix a tablespoon of vinegar, a tablespoon of glycerin, a tablespoon of coconut oil, and an egg. Blend them together until it becomes a paste form. Apply this mixture all over your scalp and leave it there for at least one hour. Then rinse your hair with shampoo. Do this every seven days.

- Tamarind and Sugarcane

Dampen tamarind with water and mix some molasses with it. Apply the mixture all over your scalp and wash it with shampoo after an hour. Do this every seven days.

Brittle Hair

First of all, you have to know that there is no treatment that will give you an overnight result. In order to treat brittle hair, you have a commitment to follow, or else you'll never get through your brittle hair dilemmas. You must follow a habit to have a better hair treatment and it is going to pay off in the end. The first thing you must do is to always wash your hair regularly. You can shampoo your hair for only once a week, but don't forget to use shampoo every day. You are also able to upturn your head while shampooing your hair in order to stimulate the blood circulation of your scalp. When you're done, dry it using the towel. Blow dryers could ruin your hair predominantly but if you really have to blow dry them, don't use it too close to your hair.

Are you aware that combing and brushing your hair can treat brittle hair? If you brush or comb your hair two times a day, it are cleaning your scalp and spreading the natural oils on your hair all over your hair. Massaging the scalp is another therapy and they are able to improve by adding some sage tea or rosemary oil. Massage your scalp and gently scratch it with your fingertips and your scalp blood flow will improve. Aside from taking good care of the hair roots, you must also look after its ends. Split ends have to be trimmed on a regular basis.

Homemade hair mask could be a great brittle hair treatment. You can make a hair mask with ripe avocado that has be crashed and combined with an egg, two tablespoon of honey, and a tablespoon of olive oil. Put on this mask all over your hair for 20 minutes every two weeks. You can also massage your scalp with amla or brahmi oil for around 15 minutes. Furthermore, are able to make a fenugreek paste by combining lemon and curd. These treatments are great for giving life to brittle hair.

Chapter 3: Making Hair Grow Faster The Natural Way

Still wondering how some women are able to grow hair faster in natural way and some women like yourself just can't do it even you think you already did everything? You must have tried using just about every kind of hair products that promise to give you the length you want to achieve instantly but just to discover that they don't actually work the way you expected!

Well, the best thing you must do is to stop using those products and try using natural treatments instead to make your hair grow fast. In this chapter you will learn some useful tips you may want to follow in order to make that mane longer and healthier.

Trim Damaged Hair

Firstly, it's important to know that you have to get rid of the damaged hairs as damaged hair can just hinder the development you've ever wanted. After that you could then let your hair grow for approximately 3 months before putting on the style of your preference. You have to remember that having wrecked hair and split ends will just lead to further damage to your locks.

Follow Natural Routines

If you're really serious about looking for the best ways of growing hair quickly the natural way, you have to be patient. Though there are other people who are ready to spend big amount of money buying hair products like conditioners, shampoos, hair cuticles, and expensive treatments, you shouldn't let yourself to be swayed by deceitful promises and

imposing commercials and ultimately follow what's trendy. Instead, just consider going for the natural regimens alone. Through that, you'll feel safer and confident using products on your hair.

Avoid Heat Treatments

Try to avoid using hair irons or blow dryers on your hair unless you're ready to have damaged hair which will hamper your hair growth. Instead, consider one of the best ways to make your hair more manageable by using natural oil treatment like coconut oil jojoba oil or olive. But you need to make sure that you're massaging the oil profoundly into your hair roots in order to infiltrate the scalp and then stimulate the development of your locks.

Get A Deep Massage For Your Head Regularly

It is recommended to get head massage right after you have applied the natural oils for your hair. Through that, you can make sure get your head blood circulation improved which could start out your hair follicles to create healthier and stronger hair strands immediately.

Get Rid Of Those Creams And Popular Medications That Never Work

You have to be careful in using those oils and creams which claim to give you fuller hair volume quickly. Most of the time, they cause more damage on your hair which could also make you spend more money in due course. Instead you should rather get rid of the dryness and damage in your hair by putting on some natural oils such as olive or coconut oil.

You'll be amazed and pleased to discover that there are treatments for your hair loss without needing to break a bank!

Chapter 4: Taking Good Care Of The Hair From The Inside And Out

Most people think that the hair doesn't have life, but this is not true. The follicle that creates the hair is actually part of the skin which is also the biggest part of the human body; thus it's openly affected by your standard of living, habits, and of course the diet.

People are always in the hunt for the best hair product that claims to repair all your hair problems without comprehending that building a healthy basis is very essential. Trying different products is not a bad thing but there are many people who don't see the fact that the wellbeing of the hair is defined by our general health.

For our body to work correctly our body needs to have specific nutritional features. For example, for the bones to keep being strong and healthy, we have to consume at least small amount of vitamin D and calcium. Here are some of good regimens you can follow in order to take care of your hair from inside and out.

Making Your Hair Glow From The Inside

1. **Riboflavin** also called **Vitamin B2** is important for the body and has to be consumed regularly as it is water soluble; it means that it's not kept within the body. Vitamin B2 has a lot of purposes and it enhances the red blood cell

production, energy metabolism, vision, enzyme reactions, skin health, and it has functions as an antioxidant. You can find this vitamin in whole grains, dairy products, nuts, eggs, fortified cereals, meat, and green vegetables.

2. **Biotin** also known as **Vitamin B5** another water soluble vitamin that you have to eat every day. It's essential for the synthesis of glycogen, fat, enzyme reactions, amino acids, DNA replication, and of course healthy hair. You can get this from nuts, yeast, soybeans, egg yolks, mushrooms, and cauliflower.

3. **Omega-3 fatty acids** and **gamma-linolenic acid** are good in making the hair healthier. Flaxseed oil and evening primrose oil are also great sources of GLA. 1-2 capsules of either oil that can also be really beneficial.

4. **Vitamins** that can make your hair grow quickly are really common and could be found in many sources. These vitamins are the following:

- **Vitamin A**: Can be found in milk, fish liver oil, peaches, meat, cheese, broccoli, eggs, cabbage, spinach, apricots, and carrots. Vitamin A helps in the the production of sebum all over the scalp.
- **Vitamin C**: Can be found in citrus fruits, tomatoes, pineapples, kiwi fruit, strawberries, potatoes, green peppers, and dark green vegetables. Vitamin C maintains healthy hair and skin.
- **Vitamin E**: Can be found in soybeans, wheat germ oil, raw seeds, cold pressed vegetable oils, green leafy vegetables, nuts, and dried beans. It helps in blood circulation in the scalp.

- **Biotin**: Can be found egg yolks, milk, whole grains, rice, liver, and brewer's yeast. Biotin promotes keratin production, which is the most important part of hair.
- Inositol: Can be found in brewer's yeast, citrus fruits, liver, and whole grains. Inositol is important in keeping the hair follicles healthy.
- **Vitamin B3** or **Niacin**: Can be found in chicken, fish, pork, meat, almonds, prawns, peas, tomatoes, beans, green vegetables, wheat products, carrots, turnips, milk, and celery. Vitamin B3 promotes the blood circulation in the scalp.
- **Vitamin B5** or **Pantothenic acid**: can be found in poultry, mushrooms, brewer's yeast, fish, whole grain cereals, whole-grain breads, milk, avocados, legumes, cheese, nuts, egg yolk, potatoes, and bananas. Vitamin B stops hair loss and graying of hair.
- **Vitamin B6** and **B12**: It can greatly found in are bell peppers and spinach. They can also be found in fish, liver, and eggs.

Making Hair Glow From The Outside

1. Egg is a natural source of protein which hair can have benefit from. Mix an egg yolk with a small amount of shampoo and let it stay for about 5 minutes. Wash thoroughly.

2. Using jojoba, olive, or sweet almond oil in massaging the hair can make your hair more beautiful. Dampen your hair and put on small amounts of the oil of your choice until the hair is completely covered. Conceal the head with a shower

cap and towel for about 30 minutes, and then wash with shampoo.

3. Homemade conditioners:

- Rub a small amount of mayonnaise on to your hair to cover it, leave it for about one hour before washing it. You will be stunned at how shiny and soft your hair will be after this, because mayonnaise can be a great source of protein.

- Use condensed milk in place of your regular conditioner. This also provides protein that gives the hair extra-special shine.

4. Mix sandalwood oil with jojoba oil, olive oil or your favorite oil, apply the mixture through your hair for instant slickness, this will rapidly control and condition brittle, unmanageable hair.

5. If you want to have a shinier hair, you could also mix a teaspoon amount of honey into four cups of warm water. After washing the hair with shampoo, put on the mixture through the hair, but don't wash it yet.

6. You can consider using aloe vera gel in place for the typical styling gels in order to keep that flyaway hair in position. Aloe vera also sets the hair naturally.

Bonus tip

It is a common fact that exercise is not just beneficial for our waistline but also for the overall health of the body and it's again essential to the health of the hair. Workout improves the health of the hair by increasing the blood circulation.

You also have to remember that smoking can also affect the hair. People that smoke are four times more possible to have gray hair compare to the people who don't. People who smoke are also more prone to hair loss.

Having healthy hair is one of the signs of overall wellbeing. You have to take care of your body all together and you'll have strong healthy hair that you will be proud of.

Chapter 5: Important Routine To Make Hair Stronger From The Roots

To fight hair loss, you must start by making your hair stronger from the roots. But how can you do this?

It is actually not as difficult as you might think it would be. There are a lot of people who are trying to repair their hair loss problems without the right knowledge on doing so. They go for anything they saw on TV that promises to fix their hair in a short period of time like hair loss pills and other treatments that are not always the best decisions to make.

Why don't you just use a simple, natural method that is proven to work to fight hair loss? In this chapter you will learn are some methods you can follow to make your hair stronger from roots to the tip, while stopping further loss of hair simultaneously.

Healthy Scalp Is Healthy Hair

The first step to conscious hair care is to understand the importance of scalp care. Diseases of the scalp and scalp issues as dandruff, psoriasis, seborrheic dermatitis of the scalp, and inadequate scalp care have a huge impact on the condition of the hair. Weakened hair roots will produce weak and thin hair. Excessive oily scalp and dandruff are the most common cause of hair loss. It can also be the cause of poor hair growth. Take care of your scalp and it will reward you by producing strong hair.

The best remedies for oily scalp are herbal lotions and rinsing hair with herbs. There are many herbs that reduce the oiliness of the scalp. For example: Horsetail, Lavender, Lemon balm, Rosemary. Herbs are completely natural and safer for the scalp than retail cosmetics which contain preservatives. Too high concentration of preservatives in the product can irritate the scalp. Some scalps may be allergic to certain preservatives, regardless of concentration.

Dry scalp needs moisturizing. You can use honey, natural yogurt, flaxseed, rinsing hair with Calendula, Sage or Parsley.

Burdock is a great ally in the fight against dandruff. With it you can get rid of dandruff very quickly. Even after a one or two uses of it.

Know Your Hair Better

Each hair and scalps are different and like different things. If one product or cosmetic works great or does not work at all for your friend's hair, it does not mean it will work the same on your hair. You need to watch your hair and learn to recognize what it likes and does not like. If you are oiling your hair with coconut oil and you don't see the results this does not mean that oiling hair is not for you. This means that this oil is not for your hair. You should look for another.

Knowing your hair better will help you to take care of your hair, save your money and save the time you spend on hair care.

Oiling Hair

Oiling hair is a long followed tradition by people (especially women) from many cultures. Oiling hair makes it softer, more satin, stronger, shinier. It is the best and a natural way to get a beautiful hair. It can be used in larger amounts for a shorter or longer period of time and then washed out. And it can be done as a leave-in treatment with smaller amount of oil.

Choosing the right oil will bring your hair the benefits. There are many different variations of natural oils or mixtures of oils with herbs and extracts. Pay attention to your scalp and hair issues and consider which oil may be appropriate for your hair's problem.

Here are some advices to help you:

- Consider the availability and price. You don't have to spend a lot of money for some popular and expensive oil. There is a risk that your hair will not like this oil. If you really want to test some oil, take a small dosage. A good carrier for oils can be: coconut, olive, sesame, sweet almond or avocado.

- Essential oil must be placed in a "base" carrier oil first. Never apply essential oils to your scalp or hair without the base. To be safe, use mix of 3-10 drops of essential oil with 1 or a few more tablespoons of carrier oil at first.

- Some scalps do not like oils. So, if you are losing hair after oiling it, stop applying it.

- If you are worried that your hair will be still greasy, wash your hair again. The washing technique has huge importance. First, wash the scalp carefully and then distribute the foam on your whole hair and massage it for a while. Oil will be washed away.

Essential Steps For Stronger Hair

The first step you can make to make your hair stronger is to simply use conditioner cream it at the ends of the hair. Some people may find this strange but it will make difference for your hair and make it look much fuller and have volume. You are able to use vinegar and sage as a way to make your hair stronger and thicker.

Have a small amount of white vinegar and mix this with sage in a container. Shake to mix it better and put the mixture on your scalp and hair.

Why You Should Avoid Commercial Shampoo?

It must be a surprise to you, but commercial shampoos don't really affect the growth of your hair. A lot of brands claim to have a secret ingredient that will do wonders to your hair, but it's not actually a secret. About 90% of all shampoo brands have the ingredient called Sodium Laureth Sulfate (SLES) - it is a strong detergent. It can dry your hair and scalp if you are washing your hair every day with shampoo with SLES. For everyday it is better to use a gentle shampoo.

Commercial shampoos also have the ingredients called silicones. Those ingredients will make your hair beautiful, silky and shiny – immediately! Silicone is responsible for those results. But it is like a cheating.

Even though this is ideal for taking off the oil and dirt from the hair, it is bad for your hair condition. This also may be the cause of a dandruff, oily scalp or hair loss. Regular use of this product will factually make your hair dry throughout the time. Make sure to only use shampoo and different other hair care products that contain only natural elements in them.

They can have saw palmetto, aloe vera, and green tea that are all amazing for your hair and wouldn't make your hair fall out.

Chapter 6: Natural Herbal Recipes For Healthy And Nourished Hair And Scalp

Hair reflects the whole condition of someone's body. A healthy hair has to stretch by approximately 30% before it breaks. A healthy body is the reflection of a healthy scalp and bouncy hair. Herbs are able to help all types of hair keep pretty and healthy. There are many natural herbs available for hair and they are known used in many countries for hundreds of years now.

Here are some of the mostly used herbal plants you can use for your hair:

Aloe Vera, Birch, Arnica, Catmint, Burdock, Horsetail, Chamomile, Marigold, Licorice, Nettles, Rosemary, Parsley, Southernwood, Sage, Chamomile, Stinging nettle, and Mulberries. Soy is also similarly important in order to prevent the hair loss.

Some of herbal rinses have the potential to help cure scalp issues such as itchy, dandruff, flaky scalp, oily scalp, stunted growth. Herbs can help with circulation in the scalp and accelerate hair growth by the stimulation of the hair follicles.

A hair rinse is a very cheap way to strengthen and treat scalp and hair.

Herbal Hair Rinses:

For hair loss and thinning: Burdock, Bhringraj, Amla, Fenugreek, Hops, Horsetail, Lavender, Nettle, Red clover, Rosemary, Sage, Shikakai, Thyme, Tulsi, Watercress, Yashtimadhu

For luster: Aloe vera, Basil, Aritha, Dandelion, Horsetail, Nettle, Parsley, Rosemary, Seaweed, Shikakai

For dry hair and scalp: Calendula, Comfrey, Flaxseed (linseed), Ginger root, Lavender, Parsley, Sage

For oily hair and scalp: Horsetail, Lavender, Lemon balm, Lemongrass, Nettle, Peppermint, Rosemary, Thyme, Watercress, Yarrow

For blond highlights: Chamomile, Mullein, Rhubarb root

For red highlights: Hibiscus, Red clover, Rose hips

For dark highlights: Black tea, Coffee, Black walnut, Cloves, Comfrey, Rosemary, Sage

Burdock root hair rinse recipe to prevent hair loss and promote hair growth

Ingredients:

A teaspoon of Burdock root
200 ml of water

Directions

Boil water together with the burdock root in a pot for ten minutes. Then let it brew under the cover for a further 20 minutes. Strain the Burdock root with a strainer. Use the liquid as a final rinse on washed hair or as a skin toner. Put the liquid into a spray bottle and spritz your scalp.

Making other herbal hair rinses is very simple. To make the Nettle or Rosemary rinse is similar to other infusions. Use a tablespoon of a herb to 300-500 ml of boiling water. Brew it under the cover for 10-15 minutes. Strain the herb with a strainer and allow the rinse to cool. Use it as a final rinse on washed and conditioned hair.

Drinking plenty of water, herbal teas, unsweetened fruit juice are also known to make your hair healthier. Nettle tea or a horsetail tea are the one of the best for hair growth. Drink it every day for 3 month. When the time is up do the break for 1 month.

Collagen that's so important for lavish hair can be found in Silica. Zine is able to boost thyroid function and lessen the chance of early hair loss which comes from underactive thyroid. The Butterfly Pea herb was known to be essential ingredient of Thai herbal medicines that cure hair loss and early grey hair. Amla is beneficial in restoring the hair's normal acid like the alkaline balance. Shikakai and Reetha are useful and effective in making the hair healthier.

Massage your scalp with warm olive oil or almond oil. Mix a half cup of water with two egg yolks, and stir well. Use the mixture to massage on your scalp and hair for about five to ten minutes. Let it on your hair a couple of minutes and rinse with lukewarm water. Rinse it again with a mixture of apple cider vinegar and clean water. If you have a very dry hair, you can use brews of elderflower, sage, or parsley. You frizzy hair will restore its natural moisture. If you have oily or greasy hair, you can rinse is with lemon balm, mint, lavender, or rosemary. You can mix lavender oil with coconut oil and boil it, when it cools down, apply it on your scalp during the night and wash it with natural shampoo the next morning.

Chapter 7: The Wealth Of Hair Products In Your Kitchen

Take a look around in your kitchen. There are many food products that you eat every day which you can use for your hair. If you can eat something, you can put it on your hair. ☺

Oils

Natural oils make the hair smooth, soft and shiny. Oiling hair do not moisturize it but prevents the moisture loss. Oil works as a natural hair cover. Also some of them have the ability to repair damaged hair: like coconut oil or palm oil. These oils penetrate deep into the hair and repair defects in the core of the hair.

You can successfully use any natural oil: olive oil, almond oil, sesame oil, walnut oil, soybean oil, avocado oil, apricot kernel oil, pumpkin seed oil, rapeseed oil, sunflower oil and many others that exist. As you can see there are plenty of oils that you can use for oiling the hair.

1-2 tablespoons is enough to cover all of the hair. If you have a short or thin hair use less oil.

Gelatine

Hair lamination treatment with gelatin is a great natural remedy for your hair. Gelatine is a source of collagen which is considered to be proteins. So, lamination treatment regenerates the hair. After the treatment, the hair is incredibly silky. This effect may persist for several days.

Recipe: Dissolve gelatin in a 1/2 cup of boiling water. Add a teaspoon of oil. Mix all the ingredients. When the mixture cools down apply it on dry hair. Wrap your hair in a towel and keep the mixture on the hair for about an hour. You can heat the towel using a hair dryer. After an hour, wash your hair.

Perform gelatin hair lamination once every 2 weeks.

Coffee

Coffee contains caffeine which stimulates hair follicles to grow. Moreover, the coffee may be naturally darkening your hair. So, if you are a blond do not rinse hair in coffee.

Brew strong coffee, drain the coffee dregs, and when it gets cold soak your scalp and hair in this liquid. Do not rinse it with water again. To see the effects of coffee you should be systematic.

Green tea

Green tea is full of vitamins (A, B1, B2, C, E, K), caffeine, essential oils, microelements (fluoride, calcium, iron, potassium, sodium, zinc). Green tea has health benefits and great influence on the hair. Similarly to coffee green tea can accelerate hair growth and strengthen the roots.

Make a pot of tea, brew it fora few minutes, and when it gets cold rinse your scalp and hair with this liquid.

Plain yogurt

It is the best for a dry and irritated scalp. Use the plain yoghurt like a mask on your scalp. Apply it on the scalp for 30 minutes and when the time is up wash your hair.

Potato flour

Teaspoon potato flour added to the hair mask will make your hair smoother and looking shinier.

Honey

Honey is rich in minerals and vitamins. It acts on the hair as a humectant. Honey attracts moisture, so better use it before washing the hair. Otherwise your hair may lose moisture and will look dry.

Add a tablespoon of honey to the mixture for the hair.

Linseed (flaxseed)

If you have a dry, curly or wavy hair the flaxseed hair gel could be a remedy for your hair.

The flaxseed hair gel can be used in several ways:

1. As a hair mask before or after washing your hair.

Put the flaxseed gel on your hair (solo or in a mixture) for about an hour. Applied after washing it does not need to be washed off with shampoo for the second time.

2. As a hair styling product.

Apply the gel to your wet hair by smoothing it on. Use more product than you normally would. Drying hair naturally you can feel stiffness. When your hair dries, knead hair with your hand. Then your curls or waves will be defined and soft.

Apple cider vinegar

Soaking in vinegar closes the hair cuticles. This helps to keep the moisture of the hair. As a result the hair will be smoother and shinier.

Add a tablespoon of apple cider vinegar to a liter of lukewarm water and rinse your hair after washing it. Do not rinse with water again.

Conclusion

Thank you again for purchasing this book!

A lot of hair care products today have chemicals that could lead to hair damage. Hairsprays have alcohol that can make the hair and scalp dry and make you have split ends. The truth is that shampoos remove the natural oils off the hair. On the whole, we normally buy hair care products because we think they improve the condition of our hair while trying to attain a specific feel and appearance. We purchase these products because we want to clean our hair. We buy them because we think they can help us in managing our hair easier. And we use them almost every day.

It's a cycle that continues and really doesn't offer any advantage to the hair. With the amount of chemical that commercial hair products can give us, you have to consider the use of natural hair care products for the hair.

All natural hair care products, especially the homemade ones, don't contain any of the harmful chemicals that a lot of commercially available hair care products we can find in the market have. The fact is that a lot of people think that natural products are not going to work better than the chemically loaded counterparts. When it comes to natural hair care products, this is not the case. The truth is that natural products normally work better since you don't need to fight the damage from chemical essences that are found in commercially products in the market. Natural hair products can clean your hair, style the hair, and even for certain kinds of deep scalp and hair treatments. For all hair care products that contain harmful chemicals, there's always a natural alternative that doesn't have these unneeded chemical extracts and additives.

Should you find this book extremely of help, sharing it with your friends and loved ones will be greatly valued.

Thank you and good luck!

Check Out My Other Books

Bellow you will find my other books that are popular on Kindle.

Health & beauty:

Body Scrubs: 30 Organic Homemade Body And Face Scrubs, The Best All-Natural Recipes For Soft, Radiant And Youthful Skin

Essential Oils Guide: The Ultimate Guide To Essential Oils For Weight Loss, Stress Relief, Aromatherapy, Beauty Care, Easy Recipes For Health & Beauty

Essential Oils For Pets: Essential Oils For Dogs: 40 Safe & Effective Therapies And Remedies To Keep Your Dog Healthy From Puppy To Adult

Anti-Aging Skin Care Secrets: Younger Skin Without Scalpel And Botox. Discover How To Rejuvenate Your Skin Quickly And Maintain A Youthful Appearance

Growing orchids:

Orchids: Growing Orchids Made Easy And Pleasant. The Most Common Errors In The Cultivation Of Orchids. Let Your Orchids Grow For Many Years

Orchids Care For Hobbyists: The Advanced Guide For Orchid Enthusiasts

Phalaenopsis Orchids Care: 30 Most Important Things To Remember When Growing Phalaenopsis Orchids, How To Give The Best Life To Your Plants

Orchids Care Bundle (Orchids + Orchids Care For Hobbyists): Growing Orchids Made Easy And Pleasant + The Advanced Guide For Orchid Enthusiasts

Phalaenopsis Orchids Box Set 2 in 1: Phalaenopsis Orchids Care + Orchids Care For Hobbyists

Orchids Care Bundle 3 in 1: Orchids + Orchids Care For Hobbyists + Phalaenopsis Orchids Care

Speed Reading Guide For Beginners:

Speed Reading Guide For Beginners: Get Your Fast
Reading Skill The Easy Way. Simple Techniques To
Increase Your Reading Speed In Less 24 Hours

You can simply search for the titles on the Amazon website
to find them.

Best regards!